RHEUMATOID ARTHRITIS RELIEF COOKBOOK

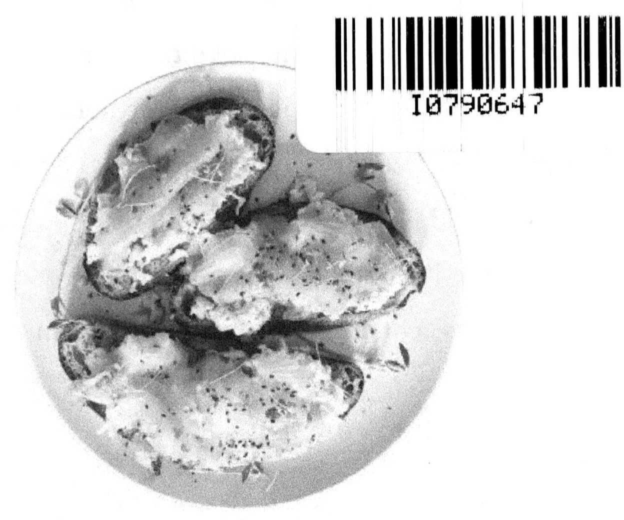

20 HEALTHY ANTI INFLAMMATORY RECIPES TO FIGHT RA

WILLIE S. HARPER

OTHER BOOKS BY THE AUTHOR

HASHIMOTO DIET FOR NEWLY DIAGNOSED RECIPE COOKBOOK

NO GALLBLADDER DIET RECIPE COOKBOOK

INSULIN RESISTANCE DIET COOKBOOK

PLANT BASED MEDITERRANEAN DIET COOKBOOK

JUICING FOR CANCER RECIPE BOOK FOR NEWLY DIAGNOSED

JUICING FOR DIABETES RECIPE BOOK

ALZHEIMER'S SOLUTION DIET COOKBOOK FOR BEGINNERS

DIVERTICULITIS DIET COOKBOOK

ACID REFLUX DIET COOKBOOK FOR BEGINNERS

AYURVEDA COOKBOOK FOR WOMEN

LOW OXALATE DIET BOOK

BARIATRIC DIET COOKBOOK

JUICING RECIPES FOR GUT HEALTH

AFIB COOKBOOK

THE AUTOIMMUNE PROTOCOL COOKBOOK

HEART HEALTHY COOKBOOK FOR BEGINNERS 2023

GOUT DIET COOKBOOK

RENAL DIET SMOOTHIE RECIPES FOR SENIORS

DIABETIC RENAL DIET COOKBOOKCIRRHOSIS DIET CONTROL COOKBOOK

TABLE OF CONTENT

Introduction: Welcome to the Rheumatoid Arthritis Relief Cookbook

Sarah used to reside in a little community tucked away among undulating hills. Sarah loved to garden and was very interested in discovering the marvels of nature. Her happiness, though, was overshadowed by rheumatoid arthritis.

Sarah endured joint discomfort and inflammation every day, which made even the smallest activities seem insurmountable. She set out on a quest to find relief and consulted experts and healers along the way. She learned the value of diet in controlling her condition during her search.

Sarah spent her time developing delectable meals that would not only delight her taste buds but also help her symptoms as a result of her discoveries. The Rheumatoid Arthritis Relief Cookbook was created; it is a compilation of twenty dishes that have been thoughtfully designed to offer solace, sustenance, and relief.

This cookbook has a wide variety of delectable foods packed with anti-inflammatory components. Each meal, from the flavorful Quinoa Salad with Turmeric to the soothing Creamy Butternut Squash Soup, is created to promote joint health and general well-being.

Join us on this gastronomic journey as we investigate the therapeutic potential of food and adopt a rheumatoid arthritis-friendly diet. Make this cookbook your go-to travel partner as you embark on your journey to a better, healthier life.

RECIPES

Recipe 1: **Anti-Inflammatory Smoothie**

- 1 cup spinach
- 1 cup pineapple chunks
- 1 small banana
- 1 tablespoon chia seeds
- 1 cup coconut water

Instructions:

1. In a blender, combine all the ingredients.
2. Blend until smooth and well combined.
3. Pour into a glass and serve immediately.

Cook Time: 5 minutes

Serving: 1

Nutritional Information: Calories: 180, Protein: 4g, Carbohydrates: 40g, Fat: 3g, Fiber: 9g

Recipe 2: **Turmeric-Spiced Quinoa Salad**

- 1 cup cooked quinoa
- 1 cup diced cucumber
- 1 cup cherry tomatoes, halved
- 1/2 cup chopped fresh parsley
- 1/4 cup diced red onion
- 2 tablespoons olive oil
- 1 tablespoon lemon juice
- 1 teaspoon ground turmeric
- Salt and pepper to taste

Instructions:

1. In a large bowl, combine the cooked quinoa, cucumber, cherry tomatoes, parsley, and red onion.
2. In a small bowl, whisk together the olive oil, lemon juice, ground turmeric, salt, and pepper.
3. Pour the dressing over the quinoa mixture and toss gently to coat.
4. Refrigerate for at least 30 minutes before serving.

Cook Time: 15 minutes (excluding quinoa cooking time)

Serving: 4

Nutritional Information: Calories: 180, Protein: 4g, Carbohydrates: 23g, Fat: 8g, Fiber: 4g

Recipe 3: **Ginger-Garlic Baked Salmon**

- 4 salmon fillets
- 2 cloves garlic, minced
- 1 tablespoon grated fresh ginger
- 2 tablespoons soy sauce
- 1 tablespoon honey
- 1 tablespoon sesame oil
- 1 tablespoon lime juice
- Salt and pepper to taste

Instructions:

1. Preheat the oven to 375°F (190°C) and line a baking dish with parchment paper.
2. In a small bowl, mix together the garlic, ginger, soy sauce, honey, sesame oil, lime juice, salt, and pepper.
3. Place the salmon fillets in the prepared baking dish and pour the marinade over them, making sure they are evenly coated.

4. Bake for 12-15 minutes or until the salmon is cooked through and flakes easily with a fork.

5. Serve hot with your choice of side dishes.

Cook Time: 15 minutes

Serving: 4

Nutritional Information: Calories: 280, Protein: 24g, Carbohydrates: 6g, Fat: 18g, Fiber: 0g

Recipe 4: **Roasted Vegetable Medley with Herbs**

- 2 cups mixed vegetables (such as bell peppers, zucchini, carrots, and broccoli), cut into bite-sized pieces
- 2 tablespoons olive oil
- 1 teaspoon dried thyme
- 1 teaspoon dried rosemary
- Salt and pepper to taste

Instructions:

1. Preheat the oven to 400°F (200°C) and line a baking sheet with parchment paper.

2. In a bowl, toss the mixed vegetables with olive oil, dried thyme, dried rosemary, salt, and pepper until evenly coated.

3. Spread the vegetables in a single layer on the prepared baking sheet.

4. Roast in the oven for 20-25 minutes or until the vegetables are tender and lightly browned, stirring once halfway through.

5. Remove from the oven and serve as a side dish or as a main course with grains or protein.

Cook Time: 25 minutes

Serving: 2

Nutritional Information: Calories: 150, Protein: 3g, Carbohydrates: 12g, Fat: 10g, Fiber: 5g

Recipe 5: Creamy Butternut Squash Soup

-   1 medium butternut squash, peeled, seeded, and cubed

-   1 onion, chopped

-   2 cloves garlic, minced

-   2 cups vegetable broth

- 1 cup coconut milk

- 1 teaspoon ground cumin

- 1/2 teaspoon ground nutmeg

- Salt and pepper to taste

- Fresh cilantro for garnish (optional)

Instructions:

1. In a large pot, sauté the chopped onion and minced garlic over medium heat until fragrant and translucent.

2. Add the cubed butternut squash, vegetable broth, coconut milk, ground cumin, ground nutmeg, salt, and pepper to the pot. Bring to a boil.

3. Reduce heat to low, cover, and simmer for 20-25 minutes or until the squash is tender and easily mashed with a fork.

4. Use an immersion blender or transfer the mixture to a blender and blend until smooth and creamy.

5. Serve hot, garnished with fresh cilantro if desired.

Cook Time: 30 minutes

Serving: 4

Nutritional Information: Calories: 180, Protein: 3g, Carbohydrates: 25g, Fat: 8g, Fiber: 5g

Recipe 6: Lemon-Tahini Kale Salad

- 4 cups chopped kale leaves
- 1/4 cup tahini
- 2 tablespoons lemon juice
- 2 tablespoons water
- 1 clove garlic, minced
- 1 tablespoon olive oil
- Salt and pepper to taste
- 1/4 cup sliced almonds, toasted (optional)

Instructions:

1. In a large bowl, combine the chopped kale leaves and set aside.

2. In a separate bowl, whisk together the tahini, lemon juice, water, minced garlic, olive oil, salt, and pepper until well combined.

3. Pour the dressing over the kale and massage it into the leaves with your hands for a few minutes to soften the kale.

4. Let the salad sit for about 10 minutes to allow the flavors to meld.

5. Sprinkle with toasted sliced almonds, if desired, before serving.

Cook Time: 10 minutes

Serving: 2

Nutritional Information: Calories: 220, Protein: 7g, Carbohydrates: 15g, Fat: 16g, Fiber: 4g

Recipe 7: **Baked Chicken Thighs with Herbs**

-   4 bone-in, skin-on chicken thighs
-   2 tablespoons olive oil
-   1 teaspoon dried thyme
-   1 teaspoon dried rosemary
-   1/2 teaspoon paprika
-   Salt and pepper to taste
-   Fresh parsley for garnish (optional)

Instructions:

1. Preheat the oven to 400°F (200°C) and line a baking sheet with foil.

2. In a small bowl, mix together the olive oil, dried thyme, dried rosemary, paprika, salt, and pepper.

3. Place the chicken thighs on the prepared baking sheet and brush them with the herb mixture, ensuring they are evenly coated.

4. Bake for 25-30 minutes or until the chicken is cooked through and the skin is crispy and golden brown.

5. Garnish with fresh parsley before serving.

Cook Time: 30 minutes

Serving: 2

Nutritional Information: Calories: 350, Protein: 24g, Carbohydrates: 0g, Fat: 28g, Fiber: 0g

Recipe 8: Cauliflower Rice Stir-Fry

- 1 head cauliflower, grated into rice-like pieces

- 1 tablespoon sesame oil

- 1/2 cup diced carrots

- 1/2 cup diced bell peppers

- 1/2 cup snap peas

- 2 cloves garlic, minced

- 2 tablespoons low-sodium soy sauce

- 1 tablespoon rice vinegar

- 1 tablespoon hoisin sauce

- 1 tablespoon chopped green onions for garnish (optional)

Instructions:

1. In a large skillet, heat the sesame oil over medium heat.

2. Add the grated cauliflower rice to the skillet and sauté for 5-7 minutes, stirring occasionally, until it becomes tender.

3. Push the cauliflower rice to one side of the skillet and add the diced carrots, bell peppers, snap peas, and minced garlic to the other side.

4. Sauté the vegetables for another 5 minutes until they are crisp-tender.

5. In a small bowl, whisk together the soy sauce, rice vinegar, and hoisin sauce.

6. Pour the sauce over the cauliflower rice and vegetables in the skillet, tossing everything together to coat evenly.

7. Cook for an additional 2-3 minutes to allow the flavors to meld.

8. Serve hot, garnished with chopped green onions if desired.

Cook Time: 20 minutes

Serving: 2

Nutritional Information: Calories: 150, Protein: 5g, Carbohydrates: 20g, Fat: 7g, Fiber: 7g

Recipe 9: Spinach and Mushroom Stuffed Bell Peppers

- 2 large bell peppers (any color), halved and seeded
- 2 cups chopped spinach
- 1 cup sliced mushrooms
- 1/2 cup cooked quinoa
- 1/4 cup diced onion
- 2 cloves garlic, minced
- 1 tablespoon olive oil
- 1/2 teaspoon dried oregano
- 1/2 teaspoon dried basil
- Salt and pepper to taste
- Grated Parmesan cheese for topping (optional)

Instructions:

1. Preheat the oven to 375°F (190°C) and line a baking dish with foil.
2. In a large skillet, heat the olive oil over medium heat.
3. Add the diced onion and minced garlic to the skillet and sauté until fragrant and translucent.
4. Add the sliced mushrooms and cook until they have released their moisture and are tender.
5. Stir in the chopped spinach, cooked quinoa, dried oregano, dried basil, salt, and pepper. Cook for an additional 2-3 minutes until the spinach has wilted.
6. Arrange the bell pepper halves in the prepared baking dish and spoon the spinach and mushroom mixture into each half.
7. Optional: Sprinkle grated Parmesan cheese on top of each stuffed bell pepper.
8. Bake for 25-30 minutes or until the bell peppers are tender and the filling is heated through.
9. Serve hot as a main course or a side dish.

Cook Time: 40 minutes (including quinoa cooking time)

Serving: 2

Nutritional Information: Calories: 180, Protein: 8g, Carbohydrates: 22g, Fat: 8g, Fiber: 6g

Recipe 10: Black Bean and Sweet Potato Chili

- 1 tablespoon olive oil
- 1 small onion, chopped
- 2 cloves garlic, minced
- 1 small sweet potato, peeled and diced
- 1 red bell pepper, diced
- 1 can (15 oz) black beans, drained and rinsed
- 1 can (14 oz) diced tomatoes
- 1 cup vegetable broth
- 1 tablespoon chili powder
- 1 teaspoon ground cumin
- 1/2 teaspoon smoked paprika
- Salt and pepper to taste
- Fresh cilantro for garnish (optional)

Instructions:

1. In a large pot, heat the olive oil over medium heat.

2. Add the chopped onion and minced garlic to the pot and sauté until fragrant and translucent.

3. Add the diced sweet potato and red bell pepper to the pot and cook for 5-7 minutes, stirring occasionally, until the sweet potato starts to soften.

4. Stir in the black beans, diced tomatoes, vegetable broth, chili powder, ground cumin, smoked paprika, salt, and pepper.

5. Bring the chili to a boil, then reduce the heat to low, cover, and simmer for 20-25 minutes, or until the sweet potato is tender.

6. Serve hot, garnished with fresh cilantro if desired.

Cook Time: 30 minutes

Serving: 4

Nutritional Information: Calories: 220, Protein: 9g, Carbohydrates: 40g, Fat: 4g, Fiber: 9g

Recipe 11: Quinoa Stuffed Portobello Mushrooms

-   4 large Portobello mushrooms
-   1 cup cooked quinoa
-   1/2 cup diced bell peppers
-   1/2 cup diced zucchini
-   1/4 cup chopped red onion
-   2 cloves garlic, minced
-   2 tablespoons olive oil
-   1 tablespoon balsamic vinegar
-   1/2 teaspoon dried thyme
-   Salt and pepper to taste
-   Grated Parmesan cheese for topping (optional)

Instructions:

1. Preheat the oven to 375°F (190°C) and line a baking sheet with parchment paper.
2. Remove the stems from the Portobello mushrooms and gently scrape out the gills using a spoon.
3. In a large skillet, heat the olive oil over medium heat.
4. Add the diced bell peppers, diced zucchini, chopped red onion, and minced garlic to the skillet. Sauté until the vegetables are tender.

5. Stir in the cooked quinoa, balsamic vinegar, dried thyme, salt, and pepper. Cook for an additional 2-3 minutes to allow the flavors to meld.

6. Place the Portobello mushrooms on the prepared baking sheet and spoon the quinoa mixture into each mushroom cap.

7. Optional: Sprinkle grated Parmesan cheese on top of each stuffed mushroom.

8. Bake for 15-20 minutes or until the mushrooms are tender and the filling is heated through.

9. Serve hot as a satisfying vegetarian main dish or a hearty side.

Cook Time: 30 minutes (including quinoa cooking time)

Serving: 4

Nutritional Information: Calories: 180, Protein: 7g, Carbohydrates: 25g, Fat: 7g, Fiber: 5g

Recipe 12: Salmon and Avocado Sushi Roll

- 4 sheets of sushi nori (seaweed)
- 2 cups cooked sushi rice

- 2 ounces smoked salmon, thinly sliced

- 1 small avocado, sliced

- 1/4 cup julienned cucumber

- Soy sauce and wasabi for serving

Instructions:

1. Place a sheet of sushi nori on a bamboo sushi mat or a clean kitchen towel.

2. Spread a thin layer of sushi rice evenly over the nori, leaving about 1 inch at the top uncovered.

3. Lay slices of smoked salmon, avocado, and julienned cucumber in a line across the center of the rice.

4. Using the sushi mat or towel, tightly roll the sushi from the bottom, applying gentle pressure to ensure it holds its shape.

5. Wet the uncovered edge of the nori with water to seal the roll.

6. Repeat the process with the remaining ingredients to make additional rolls.

7. Use a sharp knife to slice each roll into bite-sized pieces.

8. Serve the sushi rolls with soy sauce and wasabi for dipping.

Cook Time: 30 minutes (including rice cooking time)

Serving: 4

Nutritional Information: Calories: 240, Protein: 8g, Carbohydrates: 45g, Fat: 4g, Fiber: 3g

Recipe 13: Grilled Lemon-Herb Chicken Breast

- 2 boneless, skinless chicken breasts
- 2 tablespoons olive oil
- Juice of 1 lemon
- 1 teaspoon dried thyme
- 1 teaspoon dried rosemary
- Salt and pepper to taste
- Fresh parsley for garnish (optional)

Instructions:

1. Preheat the grill to medium-high heat.
2. In a small bowl, whisk together the olive oil, lemon juice, dried thyme, dried rosemary, salt, and pepper.
3. Place the chicken breasts in a shallow dish and pour the marinade over them, ensuring they are well coated.

4. Let the chicken marinate for at least 30 minutes, or up to
    overnight in the refrigerator.
5. Remove the chicken from the marinade and discard any
    excess.
6. Grill the chicken breasts for 6-8 minutes per side, or until
    cooked through and no longer pink in the center.
7. Remove from the grill and let the chicken rest for a few
    minutes before slicing.
8. Garnish with fresh parsley if desired before serving.

Cook Time: 20 minutes (including marinating time)

Serving: 2

Nutritional Information: Calories: 200, Protein: 26g,
Carbohydrates: 1g, Fat: 9g, Fiber: 0g

Recipe 14: Quinoa and Vegetable Stir-Fry

-   1 cup cooked quinoa
-   1 tablespoon olive oil
-   1/2 cup sliced carrots
-   1/2 cup sliced bell peppers
-   1/2 cup chopped broccoli florets

- 1/2 cup snap peas
- 2 cloves garlic, minced
- 2 tablespoons low-sodium soy sauce
- 1 tablespoon rice vinegar
- 1 tablespoon honey or maple syrup
- 1 tablespoon sesame seeds for garnish (optional)

Instructions:

1. In a large skillet or wok, heat the olive oil over medium-high heat.
2. Add the sliced carrots, sliced bell peppers, chopped broccoli florets, snap peas, and minced garlic to the skillet. Stir-fry for 4-5 minutes, or until the vegetables are crisp-tender.
3. In a small bowl, whisk together the soy sauce, rice vinegar, and honey or maple syrup.
4. Push the vegetables to one side of the skillet and add the cooked quinoa to the other side.
5. Pour the sauce over the quinoa and vegetables, tossing everything together to coat evenly.
6. Cook for an additional 2-3 minutes to heat everything through.
7. Serve hot, garnished with sesame seeds if desired.

Cook Time: 15 minutes (including quinoa cooking time)

Serving: 2

Nutritional Information: Calories: 250, Protein: 8g, Carbohydrates: 35g, Fat: 9g, Fiber: 6g

Recipe 15: Turmeric-Ginger Smoothie

- 1 cup unsweetened almond milk
- 1 banana
- 1/2 cup frozen pineapple chunks
- 1/2 cup frozen mango chunks
- 1-inch piece of fresh ginger, peeled
- 1/2 teaspoon ground turmeric
- 1 tablespoon honey or maple syrup (optional)

Instructions:

1. In a blender, combine the unsweetened almond milk, banana, frozen pineapple chunks, frozen mango chunks, fresh ginger, ground turmeric, and honey or maple syrup if desired.
2. Blend until smooth and creamy.

3. If the smoothie is too thick, add more almond milk until the desired consistency is reached.

4. Pour into a glass and enjoy immediately.

Preparation Time: 5 minutes

Serving: 1

Nutritional Information: Calories: 210, Protein: 3g, Carbohydrates: 52g, Fat: 2g, Fiber: 6g

Recipe 16: Lentil and Vegetable Curry

-   1 cup dried lentils,rinsed
-   2 tablespoons olive oil
-   1 small onion, chopped
-   2 cloves garlic, minced
-   1 red bell pepper, diced
-   1 zucchini, diced
-   1 carrot, diced
-   1 can (14 oz) coconut milk
-   1 can (14 oz) diced tomatoes
-   2 tablespoons curry powder
-   1 teaspoon ground cumin

- 1/2 teaspoon ground turmeric

- Salt and pepper to taste

- Fresh cilantro for garnish (optional)

Instructions:

1. Cook the lentils according to the package instructions. Drain and set aside.

2. In a large pot, heat the olive oil over medium heat.

3. Add the chopped onion and minced garlic to the pot and sauté until fragrant and translucent.

4. Add the diced red bell pepper, diced zucchini, and diced carrot to the pot. Cook for 5-7 minutes, or until the vegetables are crisp-tender.

5. Stir in the cooked lentils, coconut milk, diced tomatoes, curry powder, ground cumin, ground turmeric, salt, and pepper.

6. Bring the curry to a boil, then reduce the heat to low, cover, and simmer for 15-20 minutes to allow the flavors to meld.

7. Serve hot, garnished with fresh cilantro if desired.

8. Serve the curry over cooked basmati rice or with naan bread.

Cook Time: 45 minutes (including lentil cooking time)

Serving: 4

Nutritional Information: Calories: 320, Protein: 12g, Carbohydrates: 45g, Fat: 12g, Fiber: 12g

Recipe 17: Caprese Salad with Balsamic Glaze

-   2 large ripe tomatoes, sliced
-   8 ounces fresh mozzarella cheese, sliced
-   Fresh basil leaves
-   2 tablespoons balsamic glaze
-   Salt and pepper to taste

Instructions:

1. Arrange the tomato slices and fresh mozzarella slices on a serving platter, alternating between the two.
2. Place a fresh basil leaf on top of each tomato and mozzarella slice.
3. Drizzle the balsamic glaze over the salad.
4. Season with salt and pepper to taste.
5. Serve immediately as a refreshing appetizer or side dish.

Preparation Time: 10 minutes

Serving: 2

Nutritional Information: Calories: 220 Protein: 16g, Carbohydrates: 10g, Fat: 14g, Fiber: 2g

Recipe 18: **Greek-Style Quinoa Salad**

- 1 cup cooked quinoa
- 1 cup chopped cucumber
- 1 cup halved cherry tomatoes
- 1/2 cup crumbled feta cheese
- 1/4 cup diced red onion
- 2 tablespoons chopped Kalamata olives
- 2 tablespoons chopped fresh parsley
- 2 tablespoons lemon juice
- 1 tablespoon extra-virgin olive oil
- Salt and pepper to taste

Instructions:

1. In a large mixing bowl, combine the cooked quinoa, chopped cucumber, halved cherry tomatoes, crumbled

feta cheese, diced red onion, chopped Kalamata olives, and chopped fresh parsley.

2. In a small bowl, whisk together the lemon juice and extra-virgin olive oil.

3. Pour the dressing over the quinoa salad and toss to combine.

4. Season with salt and pepper to taste.

5. Let the salad sit for at least 15 minutes to allow the flavors to meld before serving.

6. Serve chilled as a light and refreshing side dish or as a standalone meal.

Preparation Time: 20 minutes (including quinoa cooking time)

Serving: 2

Nutritional Information: Calories: 260, Protein: 11g, Carbohydrates: 27g, Fat: 13g, Fiber: 5g

Recipe 19: Baked Lemon-Dill Salmon

- 2 salmon fillets

- 1 tablespoon olive oil

- Juice of 1 lemon
- 1 teaspoon dried dill
- Salt and pepper to taste
- Lemon wedges for serving

Instructions:

1. Preheat the oven to 375°F (190°C) and line a baking sheet with parchment paper.
2. Place the salmon fillets on the prepared baking sheet.
3. Drizzle the olive oil and lemon juice over the salmon.
4. Sprinkle the dried dill, salt, and pepper evenly over the salmon.
5. Gently rub the seasonings into the fish to ensure even coating.
6. Bake for 12-15 minutes, or until the salmon is cooked through and flakes easily with a fork.
7. Serve hot, accompanied by lemon wedges for additional flavor.

Cook Time: 15 minutes

Serving: 2

Nutritional Information: Calories: 320, Protein: 36g, Carbohydrates: 1g, Fat: 20g, Fiber: 0g

Recipe 20: Berry Chia Pudding

- 1 cup unsweetened almond milk

- 1/4 cup chia seeds

- 1 tablespoon honey or maple syrup

- 1/2 teaspoon vanilla extract

- 1 cup mixed berries (strawberries, blueberries, raspberries)

Instructions:

1. In a glass jar or bowl, combine the unsweetened almond milk, chia seeds, honey or maple syrup, and vanilla extract. Stir well to combine.
2. Let the mixture sit for 5 minutes, then stir again to prevent clumping.
3. Cover the jar or bowl and refrigerate for at least 2 hours or overnight, allowing the chia seeds to absorb the liquid and thicken into a pudding-like consistency.
4. Before serving, give the chia pudding a good stir to redistribute the chia seeds.
5. Top with mixed berries and enjoy as a healthy and satisfying breakfast or snack.

Preparation Time: 5 minutes (plus chilling time)

Serving: 2

Nutritional Information: Calories: 200, Protein: 6g, Carbohydrates: 25g, Fat: 9g, Fiber: 10g

Conclusion: Embracing a Rheumatoid Arthritis-Friendly Diet

Finally, the "Rheumatoid Arthritis Relief Cookbook" offers a selection of 20 delectable and healthy dishes that are meant to lessen the effects of rheumatoid arthritis and improve overall health. Each meal has been carefully crafted using ingredients that have been shown to have anti-inflammatory properties, making it an essential component of a rheumatoid arthritis management approach.

The recipes in this cookbook range from filling main dishes like the Quinoa Stuffed Portobello Mushrooms and Grilled Lemon-Herb Chicken Breast to light options like the Turmeric-Ginger Smoothie and Greek-Style Quinoa Salad, satisfying your palate while nourishing your body.

By including these meals into your normal mealtime routine, you may use food's therapeutic properties as a natural remedy for treating the signs and symptoms of rheumatoid arthritis.

Whether you're searching for relief from joint pain, inflammation, or general discomfort, these dishes provide a delicious and enjoyable way to support your health journey.

Bid adieu to bland and uninspiring meals and hello to a culinary adventure that prioritizes taste and wellness. Utilizing the "Rheumatoid Arthritis Relief Cookbook," you may manage your rheumatoid arthritis while still enjoying every bite. Happy and healthy greetings to you!

www.ingramcontent.com/pod-product-compliance
Lightning Source LLC
Chambersburg PA
CBHW061546250726
48657CB00006B/2318